Pharmacy Technician Certification Guide

Examination Workbook

Mark Greenwald, RPh.

PharmacyTrainer, Inc.

Copyright Information

Pharmacy Technician Certification Guide, Examination Workbook

ISBN: **0-9856895-5-2**
ISBN-13:   **978-0-9856895-5-1**

Proudly printed in the United States of America

PharmacyTrainer, Inc.
2135 N Roxbury Rd
Avon Park, FL 33825

http://PharmacyTrainer.com

Table of Contents

PharmacyTrainer™
Pharmacy Technician Certification Review
Examination Workbook

A Brief Introduction

Thank you for purchasing our Examination Workbook! This book is designed to be used with the *PharmacyTrainer Pharmacy Technician Certification Guide* textbook. By using this workbook, you will be able to gauge your learning progress and identify potential weak areas that you may have.

In order to allow constant feedback, this book is divided into a number of section and math tests as well as two practice final examinations. This allows you to test your knowledge throughout your studies. This is critical in order to allow you to pinpoint problems in your study habits. Different study times and environments work for different people. You must find the combination that works best for you.

These tests are designed to be used at certain times in the reading, and a schedule is provided for you to follow. Do not skip tests or try to take them before they are due to be taken.

Section tests contain fifty questions, but they do not contain any math calculations. They may, however, contain questions on math theory. You will not need a calculator to complete a section test. Math tests are fifteen questions long. All math test questions involve calculations. You will need a calculator for these tests. Final examinations are ninety questions long and they contain math calculations. Keep your calculator handy!

I would suggest that, rather than writing in the book, you use a separate piece of paper for an answer sheet. By doing this, you are able to repeat the tests multiple times and as often as you like. Answer keys to all tests are provided in this book.

In addition to these tests, I would suggest that you employ some sort of system to learn important facts about the most commonly prescribed drugs. I have always found flash cards to be the best method. You can make your own cards, or purchase a quality set such as the PharmacyTrainer Top 200 Drug Flash Cards that are available at www.PharmacyTrainer.com.

Take your time. Study hard. It is your commitment that will make you successful both in your certification examination and in your future career as a Certified Pharmacy Technician!

Examination Schedule

As I mentioned earlier, the tests in this workbook are designed to be taken at specific times in your studies. Here is when the tests should be taken:

- ➢ **Section Test Number One**
  Take Section Test Number One after you are finished with Chapter 13
  Includes Chapters 1 thru 13

- ➢ **Math Test Number One**
  Take Math Test Number One after you complete Section Test Number One
  Includes Math contained in Chapters 19 thru 23

- ➢ **Section Test Number Two**
  Take Section Test Number Two after you are finished with Chapter 28
  Includes Chapters 14 thru 28

- ➢ **Math Test Number Two**
  Take Math Test Number One after you are finished with Chapter 31
  Includes Math contained in Chapters 21 thru 30

- ➢ **Section Test Number Three**
  Take Section Test Number Three after you are finished with Chapter 36
  Includes Chapters 29 thru 36

- ➢ **Math Test Number Three**
  Take Math Test Number One after you complete Section Test Number Three
  Includes Math contained in Chapters 33 thru 35

- ➢ **Section Test Number Four**
  Take Section Test Number Four after you are finished with Chapter 46
  Includes Chapters 37 thru 46

- ➢ **Section Test Number Five**
  Take Section Test Number Four after you are finished with Chapter 52
  Includes Chapters 47 thru 52

Section Test Number One

1. The agency charged with the approval to market new drug entities is the:
   a. US Patent Office
   b. FDA
   c. DEA
   d. State Board of Pharmacy

2. Responsibilities of the FDA include all of the following except:
   a. regulating package units
   b. regulating drug advertising
   c. issuing recalls when necessary
   d. approving patent applications

3. The agency which licenses the pharmacy is the:
   a. FDA
   b. State Board of Pharmacy
   c. State Legislators
   d. all of the above must approve the license

4. The "rules" governing the practice of pharmacy in a state are known as the:
   a. Pharmacy Practice Act
   b. Standard of Practice
   c. Administrative Code
   d. Standard Operating Procedure

5. Who are you most likely to see conducting a routine inspection of your pharmacy?
   a. a DEA investigator
   b. an FDA investigator
   c. a State Pharmacy Compliance Officer
   d. a State Police investigator

6. Usually a state will have 3 pieces of legislation governing the practice of pharmacy. Which of these is not one of them?
   a. Pharmacy Practice Act
   b. Administrative Code
   c. State Controlled Substances Act
   d. State Patented Drug Act

7. The federal DEA has jurisdiction on any:
   a. legend drug(s) within the state
   b. controlled substances within the state
   c. legend drugs that have crossed state lines
   d. controlled substances which have crossed state lines

8. True or False: it is possible for a drug to be defined as a controlled substance within your state if it doesn't appear on a federal DEA controlled substance schedule.
   a. True
   b. False

9. The governing body of pharmacy within the State is known as the:
   a. Pharmacy Committee
   b. Board of Pharmacy
   c. Governor's Pharmacy Committee
   d. State Legislature

10. The first piece of legislation which covered the purity of drugs was the:
    a. Federal Food and Drug Act
    b. Federal Food, Drug, and Cosmetic act
    c. Durham-Humphrey Amendment
    d. Kefauver-Harris Amendment

11. A bottle that contained Dyazide but was labeled Diabeta would be said to be:
    a. Adulterated
    b. misbranded
    c. both
    d. none

12. The federal Food, Drug, and Cosmetic Act was important for the fact that it was the first legislation to demand:
    a. purity of product
    b. safety of product
    c. effectiveness of product
    d. all of the above

13. Durham-Humphrey and Kefauver-Harris are both amendments of the:
    a. Federal Food and Drug Act
    b. Federal Food, Drug, and Cosmetic Act
    c. Federal Controlled Substances Act
    d. none of the above

14. Which of the following created the class known as "legend drugs"?
    a. Durham - Humphrey
    b. Kefauver - Harris
    c. Federal FDCA
    d. none of the above

15. Which of the following demanded proof of effectiveness before a new drug could be manufactured?
    a. Durham-Humphrey
    b. Kefauver-Harris
    c. Federal FDCA
    d. none of the above

16. The first attempt at controlling narcotics involved the use of:
    a. 5 "schedules"
    b. taxation
    c. a DEA license
    d. narcotics police

17. Pharmacy laws can be enacted by:
    a. the local government
    b. the state government
    c. the federal government
    d. all of the above

18. The level to which a practitioner is expected to perform is called the:
    a. Standard of Practice
    b. Pharmacy Standard
    c. Universal Requirement
    d. none of the above

19. The organization involved in certifying institutional health care organizations is called:
    a. MAACO
    b. AMOCO
    c. TJC
    d. EIEIO

20. Possible causes for a violation on a 3rd party audit would be all except:
    a. wrong pack size billed
    b. no patient signature on file
    c. wrong quantity billed
    d. all of the above would be violations

21. The NDA is used to:
    a. approve a new drug product for sale
    b. transport an investigational drug across state lines
    c. patent a drug
    d. all of the above

22. The IND is used to:
    a. approve a new drug product for sale
    b. transport an investigational drug across state lines
    c. patent a drug
    d. all of the above

23. In order to get an approval on an NDA, the applicant would need to show:
I. safety of the drug
II. effectiveness of the drug
III. proper labeling of the drug
IV. proper manufacturing conditions for the drug
    a. I and II only
    b. I and III only
    c. I, II, and IV only
    d. I, II, III, and IV

24. True or false: The same drug may be sold under more than one trade name.
    a. True
    b. False

25. The name that is used in a clinical journal will be the:
    a. chemical name
    b. generic name
    c. trade name
    d. clinical name

26. AMPI25016 would probably be an example of a(n):
    a. chemical name
    b. generic name
    c. mnemonic name
    d. abbreviation

27. The abbreviation INH stands for:
    a. ibuprofen
    b. indapamide
    c. isoniazid
    d. intal

28. In the abbreviation D5NS, what is the concentration of sugar?
    a. 5%
    b. 0.5%
    c. 0.9%
    d. 0.45%

29. Which is correct?
    a. a patent gives the right to make a product
    b. the patent runs for 15 years with a possible 5 year extension
    c. a patent forbids other US manufacturers from producing the same product
    d. you may not trademark a name

30. Which is false about a DEA number?
    a. It can be issued to a business
    b. It is a series of 2 letters and 7 numbers
    c. The first letter for a veterinarian will be a "V"
    d. The second letter should be the first letter of the practitioner's last name

31. The current system of handling controlled substances is a(n) _____ system.
    a. open
    b. closed
    c. inventory
    d. absolute

32. You receive a prescription from Dr. Goodguy for a controlled substance. The DEA number written by the doctor is AG7266908. You should:
    a. fill the prescription and ready it for the final check by the pharmacist
    b. alert the pharmacist about a problem with the DEA number verification

33. The contents of which schedule have no accepted medical use?
   a. schedule A
   b. schedule B
   c. schedule I
   d. schedule V

34. Cocaine is a member of which schedule?
   a. schedule I
   b. schedule II
   c. schedule III
   d. schedule IV

35. Which of the following may be a breach of patient confidentiality?
   a. speaking of patient specific matters in a crowded elevator
   b. discussing patient care with a coworker who is not involved in that patient's care
   c. discarding patient drug labels in the general trash
   d. all of the above

36. Which schedule would contain drugs with the lowest potential for abuse?
   a. Schedule I
   b. Schedule III
   c. Schedule V
   d. none of the schedules contain drugs with a low potential for abuse

37. When dispensing a controlled substance prescription in a retail store, what must appear on the label?
   a. the symbol "Rx only"
   b. the statement "Caution: Federal law prohibits dispensing without a prescription"
   d. the statement, "Caution: Federal law prohibits the transfer of this drug to any person other than the person for whom it was prescribed"
   e. all of the above

38. When looking at a manufacturers stock bottle, you can tell a drug is a controlled substance because of the:
   a. statement which reads: "Caution: Federal law prohibits dispensing without a prescription"
   b. statement that says: "Caution: controlled drug"
   c. the symbol "C" followed by the number of the schedule to which it belongs
   d. none of the above

39. Route of Administration refers to the:
   a. way a drug enters the body
   b. way a drug is metabolized
   c. way a prescription is dispensed
   d. type of supervision in the pharmacy

40. Which of the following pieces of legislation require that we keep pseudoephedrine behind the pharmacy counter?
    a. CSA
    b. FFDCA
    c. HIPAA
    d. CMEA

41. Which would not be an appropriate route for a drug which is extremely irritating to the stomach?
    a. a PO enteric coated tablet
    b. IM
    c. NG
    d. IV

42. Why must the route of administration be written on the drug order?
    a. Some drugs come in different forms for different routes of administration
    b. to know if the drug has to be ordered
    c. The Joint Commission requires it
    d. none of the above

43. The DSHEA legislation was passed to regulate:
    a. dietary supplements
    b. vaccines
    c. Sterile products
    d. legend drugs

44. A cream is a _____ dosage form.
    a. solid
    b. semi-solid
    c. liquid
    d. compounded

45. A patient who cannot have products containing alcohol should not take a(n):
    a. solution
    b. suspension
    c. syrup
    d. elixir

46. A drug product which consists of drug product dissolved in oil droplets that are suspended in a water based vehicle is called an:
    a. suspension
    b. solution
    c. emulsion
    d. tincture

47. In a phase I clinical trial, the investigators are testing an applicant drug's:
    a. effectiveness
    b. maximum tolerated dose
    c. appropriate dosing for the disease for which it is intended
    d. none of the above

48. NDA phase IV testing of an applicant drug takes place:
    a. before a patent is applied for
    b. before clinical trials may commence
    c. after NDA approval is given and the drug is marketed
    d. none of the above

49. Which of the following is not a requirement for establishing a pharmacy?
    a. a large break room for employees
    b. adequate storage space
    c. adequate security
    d. adequate reference materials

50. In the NDC number 00087-6071-11, the number 00087 indicates the:
    a. manufacturer of the drug
    b. name of the drug
    c. package size
    d. cost of the drug

Math Test Number One

1. The roman numeral CXXIV would be:
	a. 116
	b. 126
	c. 124
	d. 135

2. 1/3 + ½ =
	a. 2/5
	b. 3/6
	c. 5/6
	d. ¼

3. ¾ x 1/8 =
	a. 4/8
	b. 3/32
	c. 16/12
	d. 4/12

4. ¾ ÷ 1/8 =
	a. 24/4
	b. 3/32
	c. 7/8
	d. 16/8

5. Round the number 14.3648 to the nearest hundredth.
	a. 14.365
	b. 14.364
	c. 14.37
	d. 14.36

6. How many liters are contained in 46oz?
	a. 1.38
	b. 2.76
	c. 3.01
	d. 4.60

7. A person weighs 110kg. What does he weigh in pounds?
	a. 50
	b. 121
	c. 242
	d. 300

8. A child weighs 10kg. What does he weigh in pounds?
	a. 22.0
	b. 4.5
	c. 8.3
	d. 16.8

9. Write the number 254 in roman numerals.
   a. CCLIV
   b. CCIVL
   c. CCVIL
   d. CCLVI

10. Drug "B" costs $35.95 for 100ml of solution. How much would ½ a liter cost us?
    a. $86.59
    b. $98.32
    c. $179.75
    d. $84.68

11. Drug "A" costs $15.95 for 30g. What is the cost for 83g?
    a. $44.13
    b. $60.92
    c. $36.44
    d. $23.99

12. Drug "C" costs $29.95 for #100 capsules. What will #15 cost us?
    a. 4.49
    b. 3.88
    c. 2.91
    d. 6.83

13. An oral liquid costs $143.99 for 1 pint. How much would 45ml cost us?
    a. $43.28
    b. $36.19
    c. $13.50
    d. $10.33

14. If #1000 tablets cost us $69.19, how many can we buy for $6.00?
    a. 50
    b. 86
    c. 103
    d. 129

15. An ointment costs $49.56 for 45g. How much would 1 ounce cost us?
    a. $14.58
    b. $19.99
    c. $25.99
    d. $33.04

Section Test Number Two

1. Which of the following must appear on a retail prescription for a controlled substance, but not on an MAR?
    a. the prescriber's DEA number
    b. the drug name
    c. the prescriber's name
    d. the strength of the drug

2. When a drug order is telephoned to the pharmacy, the first task that must be done is to:
    a. check if the item is in stock
    b. enter the patient's information into the computer
    c. inform the caller that prescription orders may never be called in
    d. generate a "hard copy" of the prescription - write it down

3. What is a doctor's NPI number used for?
    a. ordering controlled substances
    b. ordering hypodermic supplies
    c. billing insurance claims
    d. operating an ATM machine

4. True or False: A schedule II prescription may not be transmitted by telephone under any circumstances
    a. True
    b. False

5. Which of the following appears on a hospital MAR, but not on a retail prescription?
    a. the patients billing number
    b. the patient's name
    c. the prescriber's name
    d. the drug strength

6. Which of the following will not appear on an MAR?
    a. the prescriber's name
    b. a patient billing number
    c. the patient's home address
    d. the patient's date of birth

7. How should the following appear on the label? 2gtt OU QID
    a. use 2 drops in both eyes 4 times daily
    b. use 2 drops in both ears 4 times daily
    c. use 2 drops in the right eye 4 times daily
    d. use 2 drops in the right ear 4 times daily

FOR QUESTIONS 8 and 9:
AMOXIL 125mg/5ml suspension
4ml PO TID x 10d

8. How many ml would be required to complete the therapy?
    a. 80ml
    b. 120ml
    c. 160ml
    d. 180ml

9. What instructions should appear on the label?
    a. Give 1 teaspoonful by mouth twice daily for 10 days
    b. Give 4ml by mouth twice daily for 10 days
    c. Give 4ml by mouth three times daily for 10 days
    d. Give 4ml by mouth four times daily for 10 days

10. A prescription for a schedule IV controlled substance may be written for a maximum of:
    a. 6 refills within a 12 month period
    b. 6 refills within a 6 month period
    c. 5 refills within a 12 month period
    d. 5 refills within a 6 month period

11. A prescription for 60 of a schedule II medication is presented to you. Upon checking your inventory, you find that you have only 30 in stock. You may legally:
    a. fill the 30 you have now, then fill the rest within 6 months from the date written
    b. tell the patient you must wait until you have the whole amount in stock
    c. fill the prescription for the 30 you have now, then fill for the rest if they arrive within the next 72 hours
    d. none of the above

12. Which of the following is incorrect?
    a. qhs = every bedtime
    b. ac = with food
    c. ung = ointment
    d. qs = quantity sufficient

13. Which of the following drug storage areas are not under pharmacy supervision?
    a. the cart
    b. the floor stock
    c. the crash carts
    d. none of the above

14. When a hospital nurse gives a dose of a medication, the information will be logged on the:
    a. prescription
    b. chart
    c. MAR
    d. doctor's notes

15. A hospital order states: Lotrisone cream - apply a thin layer to the diaper area 0800, 1400, 2000. This order will most likely be dispensed as:
    a. a unit dose item
    b. a bulk drug
    c. a compounded drug
    d. a non-formulary drug

16. During an inspection, an expired ampule of sodium bicarbonate injection is found in a CCU crash cart. Who will most likely be charged with the violation?
    a. the pharmacy
    b. the nursing supervisor
    c. the chief resident
    d. housekeeping

17. When working in the pharmacy, units of weight are most commonly expressed in the _____ system.
    a. avoidupois
    b. apothecary
    c. metric
    d. household

18. The unit which describes the number of positively charged ions in a liter of a salt solution is the:
    a. scruple
    b. milliequivalent
    c. dram
    d. grain

19. A microgram is one-_____ of a gram
    a. tenth
    b. hundredth
    c. thousandth
    d. millionth

20. Which of the following is incorrect?
    a. 1 tsp = 15 ml
    b. 1 oz = 30 ml
    c. 1 pt = 473 ml
    d. 1 G = 3840 ml

21. When placing weights on a pharmacy torsion balance:
    a. the weights should be gently placed in the center of the right pan, with the fingers
    b. the weights should be placed in the left pan, and the sample in the right
    c. you should never touch the weights
    d. you must zero the balance after placing the weights in the center of the right pan

22. If you need to measure a volume of 24ml, the appropriate size graduated cylinder to use is a ____ oz cylinder.
    a. 1
    b. 2

c. 4

d. 8

23. When reading the volume of liquid in a plastic graduated cylinder, the proper place to take the reading is at the:

    a. top of the meniscus

    b. bottom of the meniscus

    c. middle of the meniscus

    d. there will be no meniscus

24. Which of the following is exempt from the PPPA?

    a. atenolol SL

    b. nitroglycerin SL

    c. nifedipine SL

    d. none of the above

25. Which of the following can adversely affect the stability of prescription medications?

    a. humidity

    b. heat

    c. light

    d. all of the above

26. Compounding which is done by following a written protocol for a single patient is called:

    a. extemporaneous compounding

    b. bulk compounding

    c. bulk manufacturing

    d. none of the above

27. A package insert must be dispensed with which of the following products?

    a. amiodarone

    b. methotrexate

    c. methylphenidate

    d. conjugated estrogens

28. A prescription bottle is made of amber colored plastic or glass in order to:

    a. hide the size of the pills

    b. protect the contents from moisture

    c. protect the contents from light

    d. all of the above

29. A unit dose medication going to the nursing unit, to supplement until the cart exchange occurs, must be labeled with all of the following, except:

    a. the patient's name

    b. the patient's room number or location

    c. the drug name

    d. the schedule of administration

30. Which of the following is the best reason for ordering pharmaceuticals from your company warehouse rather than a secondary wholesaler?
    a. the purity of product is better assured
    b. a greater profit potential is available
    c. the proper storage conditions can be better assured
    d. a 222 form is not required

31. Which of the following is not required to be on a retail prescription label?
    a. the patient's name
    b. the patient's date of birth
    c. the prescriber's name
    d. the drug name

32. In an IV of D5NS, the strength of the salt solution is:
    a. 5%
    b. 0.5%
    c. 9%
    d. 0.9%

33. When prepared, an IV of sodium nitroprusside should be:
    a. run through an arterial port
    b. hung by a cardiac resident only
    c. immediately wrapped in foil
    d. frozen

34. Which of the following is true?
    a. LR = last rate used
    b. D5W contains no sugar
    c. NS contains no salt
    d. D5 1/2NS contains salt and sugar

35. OBRA requires the performance of which of the following?
    a. prospective DUR
    b. retrospective DUR
    c. education
    d. all of the above

36. The purpose of the OBRA legislation is to:
    a. save the taxpayers money
    b. upgrade the profession of pharmacy
    c. override the insurance companies
    d. all of the above

37. A prospective DUR will check for all of the following, except
    a. prescription duplication
    b. drug/drug interactions
    c. a practitioner's prescribing pattern
    d. incorrect dosages

38. OBRA requires:
    a. we counsel every customer picking up the prescription
    b. we counsel every medicare patient picking up a prescription
    c. we offer to counsel every patient picking up a prescription
    d. we offer to counsel every medicaid patient picking up a prescription

39. Who is required to conduct a retrospective DUR under the OBRA law?
    a. pharmacist
    b. state medicaid program
    c. doctor
    d. all of the above

40. In order to prove compliance with OBRA, the pharmacy must maintain:
    a. invoices
    b. written documentation
    c. insurance cards
    d. an insurance database

41. when measuring liquid in a syringe, you should read the volume indicated by the:
    a. black ring closest to the tip
    b. black ring furthest from the tip
    c. space between the two black rings
    d. none of the above

42. The smallest weight which should be measured on a pharmacy torsion balance is:
    a. 3 mg
    b. 6 mg
    c. 10 mg
    d. 12 mg

43. The process known as "stock rotation" includes the:
    a. placement of newly received product in the front of the shelf to assure that fresh stock is always available
    b. placement of newly received product in the back of the shelf to assure that old stock is used first
    c. changing the drugs that are stocked in the pharmacy to meet the changing needs of the community
    d. none of the above

44. Invoices for schedule III through V controlled substances should be filed:
    a. with your schedule II invoices
    b. with your non-controlled invoices, but separate from your schedule II invoices
    c. separate from both your schedule II invoices and your non-controlled invoices
    d. invoices do not need to be retained by the pharmacy once all the product has been checked in, and there are no shortages

45. A controlled substance in schedule II may be ordered using a:
    a. telxxon
    b. computer
    c. FDA form 222
    d. DEA form 222

46. A paper 222 form may be signed by:
    a. any pharmacist on duty
    b. only the person who signed the DEA application
    c. the person who signed the DEA application or someone holding their power of attorney
    d. the technician who will be receiving the drugs

47. Which is correct regarding the paper 222 form?
    a. copy 1 is blue and goes to the DEA
    b. copy 2 is brown and goes to the supplier
    c. copy 3 is blue and is retained by the ordering pharmacy
    d. copy 4 is yellow and gets filed with the invoice in the pharmacy

48. When completing a paper 222 form, you write the supplier's address incorrectly. You must now:
    a. discard the form in the trash and start a new form
    b. write "void" across the face of the 222, file it with your completed 222's, and start a new form
    c. draw a line through the incorrect information, initial it, and correctly write the information in the remaining space
    d use a product like "white out" to correct the information, and continue filling out the form

49. When an order containing schedule III through V drugs comes into the pharmacy, what will serve as proof of receipt?
    a. a supplier's invoice signed and dated by the pharmacist
    b. a completed 222 form
    c. a completed receipt of narcotics form
    d. any of the above

50. Any shortage of controlled substances, which cannot be rectified by the supplier, must be reported immediately to the:
    a. FDA
    b. state better business bureau
    c. DEA
    d. all of the above

Math Test Number Two

1. Convert 53° C to °F
   a. 127.4°
   b. 56.3°
   c. 82.9°
   d. 99.4°

2. Convert 79° F to °C
   a. 36.2°
   b. 59.4°
   c. 26.1°
   d. 13.7°

3. 43g of Drug "A" is added to enough sweetened vehicle to equal a final volume of 300ml. Calculate the resulting percent strength of Drug "A".
   a. 14.3
   b. 39.4
   c. 28.6
   d. 7.4

4. How much KCl would be needed to make 500ml of an 8% solution?
   a. 20g
   b. 10g
   c. 40g
   d. 80g

5. How much hydrocortisone powder would be needed to make 120g of a 10% cream?
   a. 1.2g
   b. 12g
   c. 6g
   d. 3g

6. 10ml of glycerin is dissolved in enough water to make 240ml of final solution. What is the resulting percent strength of glycerin?
   a. 2.1
   b. 8.4
   c. 10.1
   d. 4.2

7. An order states to give 2mg of epinephrine. You have a bottle of a 1:100 dilution. How much should you draw up into a syringe to give the requested dose?
   a. 0.02ml
   b. 0.20ml
   c. 2.00ml
   d. 20.00ml

8. An order calls for 160g of 15% hydrocortisone cream is written. Your pharmacy stocks hydrocortisone cream in strengths of 2% and 20%. How much of the 2% will need to be mixed with 20% to yield the final strength?

a. 44.4g
b 115.6g
c. 32.1g
d. 15.8g

9. How much 9% cream must be mixed with a 1% cream to yield 60g of a 5% cream?
    a. 3g
    b. 5g
    c. 30g
    d. 10g

10. HCTZ 25mg costs us $26.95 for a bottle of 1000 tablets. How much does 30 tabs cost us?
    a. $0.81
    b. $3.48
    c. $1.62
    d. $0.55

11. Our pharmacy uses a markup of 28% and a dispensing fee of $3.50. Drug "A" costs us $29.99 for 100g. What would our selling price be for 60g?
    a. $18.88
    b. $21.49
    c. $23.03
    d. $26.53

12. Drug "B" costs us $183.99 for 100 tablets. Dr. Strangeone writes a prescription for 30 tablets. Our pharmacy's markup is 33%, and our dispensing fee is $4.25. Calculate our selling price for the prescription.
    a. $73.42
    b. $77.67
    c. $98.63
    d. $114.65

13. A third party plan calls for reimbursement at a rate of AWP less 3% plus a dispensing fee of $4.00. The drug order calls for 15g of a cream who's AWP is $49.50 for a 60g tube. If the patient has a $5.00 copay, what will be the price the insurance company will owe us?
    a. $12.38
    b. $12.01
    c. $16.01
    d. $11.01

14. Our pharmacy uses a markup of 23%. Our dispensing fee is $3.75. The drug ordered costs us $63.19 for 100 tablets. The prescription calls for 30 tablets. What should our selling price be?

        a. $22.71
        b. $23.32
        c. $27.07
        d. $29.58

15. Our pharmacy accepts the "XYZ" prescription plan. It reimburses for prescriptions at the rate of AWP less 15% plus a dispensing fee of $4.75. The drug's AWP is $29.99 for 10 capsules. What would our total price be for a prescription that calls for 50 capsules?

        a. $132.21
        b. $127.46
        c. $119.91
        d. $148.15

Section Test Number Three

1. Which of the following calculates a pediatric dose based on the child's weight?
   - a. Young's rule
   - b. Clark's rule
   - c. Herman's rule
   - d. Levonjie's rule

2. Flow rate is a function of:
   - a. weight and volume
   - b. weight and time
   - c. volume and time
   - d. none of the above

3. Regarding °C vs. °F:
   - a. °C is always higher than °F for the same temperature value
   - b. °C is always lower than °F for the same temperature value
   - c. °C = °F
   - d. none of the above

4. When calculating % w/v, the percentage refers to the:
   - a. g/L
   - b. g/ml
   - c. g/100ml
   - d. mg/100L

5. When compounding a 20% cream using a 90% and a 5% formulation of the same cream, you would use a calculation known as:
   - a. a conversion factor
   - b. a proportion
   - c. a reduction factor
   - d. an alligation

6. True or False: A 1:100 concentration contains 10mg per 100ml
   - a. True
   - b. False

7. A person, group, or organization, other than the patient, who pays for the patient's prescription is called a:
   - a. third party payer
   - b. designated payer
   - c. unwitting payer
   - d. none of the above

8. Cost + _____ + _____ = selling price
    a. insurance fee, uncontrollable costs
    b. markup, dispensing fee
    c. AWP, insurance fee
    d. none of the above

9. Most insurance contracts call for the reimbursement of prescriptions based on a formula of:
    a. AWP ± % + dispensing fee = selling price
    b. cost + markup + dispensing fee = selling price
    c. non-controllable expenses + controllable expenses = selling price
    d. none of the above

10. A customer returns a bottle which contains 10 Dyazide capsules to your retail pharmacy. The bottle originally contained 100 capsules, and the patient says the doctor took him off the medicine. What can you do with these capsules?
    a. return them to stock in your inventory
    b. discard them immediately in the appropriate manner
    c. send them back to the wholesaler for credit and reuse
    d. none of the above

11. Two unit dose capsules of Dyazide come back to the hospital pharmacy with an order that states to D/C the medicine. What can you do with the medicine?
    a. return them to stock in your inventory
    b. discard them immediately in the appropriate manner
    c. send them back to the wholesaler for credit and reuse
    d. none of the above

12. A class II recall is appropriate when the risk of serious injury or death is:
    a. likely
    b. certain
    c. unlikely
    d. none of the above

13. Our company manufactures 125mg Drug "A" tablets in bottles of 1000. During the investigation of a customer complaint, we learn that it is likely all bottles in lot number 53287 contained only 950 tablets. When we notify the FDA of the situation, they may authorize a _____ recall.
    a. class I
    b. class II
    c. class III
    d. class IV

14. True or False: Return of an expired schedule II medication, to an authorized return center, requires the use of a 222 form.
    a. True
    b. False

15. Which of the following syringe & needle combinations has the largest diameter needle?
    a. 3ml25g1"
    b. 3ml25g1&1/2"
    c. 5ml25g2"
    d. they are all the same diameter

16. The process of assuring sterility through our actions is called:
    a. aseptic technique
    b. clean procedures
    c. conscientious activities
    d. none of the above

17. The greatest contaminant during aseptic procedures is:
    a. the HEPA filter
    b. the syringe
    c. the medication vial
    d. the person performing the work

18. A laminar flow hood works by:
    a. irradiating bacteria in the workspace
    b. blowing columns of filtered air over the workspace
    c. providing a vacuum containment of bacteria
    d. using bottled Xenon gas

19. A laminar flow hood should be professionally serviced every:
    a. 3 months
    b. 6 months
    c. 1 year
    d. 2 years

20. Which of the following is true regarding the cleaning of a laminar flow hood?
    a. the HEPA filter should be sprayed with alcohol daily
    b. wiping should be done from the bottom up and from front to back of the hood
    c. wiping should be done from the top down and from the back of the hood forward
    d. none of the above

21. Masks, gowns, and eye shields are examples of:
    a. personal protective equipment
    b. IV equipment
    c. contamination gear
    d. none of the above

22. PPE is helpful in protecting the:
    a. patient
    b. worker
    c. both
    d. neither

23. A small area of "oozing" is noticed on the HEPA filter in your hood. You should:
    a. spray the filter with alcohol
    b. wipe the area with a sterile, lint free, cloth

c. inform the pharmacist immediately
d. all of the above

24. An indication of the HEPA filter's function is:
    a. the measurement of the air flow rate at various spots within the hood
    b. the water flow rate within the filter
    c. the sound of the blower
    d. none of the above

25. A filter used in an IV line should be able to filter out particles as small as:
    a. 0.01 microns
    b. 0.22 microns
    c. 0.33 microns
    d. 0.4 microns

26. When the supplier of a schedule II controlled substance is out of stock on an item you have ordered on a 222 form, the supplier can ship the drug up to _____ days later, when the drug is back in stock.
    a. 3
    b. 30
    c. 60
    d. 120

27. What must be written on the third copy of the paper 222 form when you receive the medications you have ordered?
    I. the date
    II. the number of packages received
    III. The number of tablets, ml, or capsules received
    IV. the pharmacist's initials on each line and signature on the face

    a. I, III, & IV only
    b. I, II, & IV only
    c. I & IV only
    d. I, II, III, & IV

28. What will decrease the expiration date on an injectable multi-dose vial from the manufacturer's date on the package?
    a. storage according to the label directions
    b. storage in a floor stock area
    c. puncture with a needle
    d. all of the above

29. Before withdrawing medicine from a multi-use vial, you must:
    a. swab the needle with alcohol
    b. swab the rubber stopper with alcohol
    c. swab the counter with alcohol
    d. all of the above

30. Controlled substances may be kept in stock by:
    a. keeping them together in a locked cabinet
    b. keeping them together on a back shelf

  c. keeping them together in a spot under the counter
  d. any of the above options

31. The temperature scale used in the field of science is the _____ scale.
  a. fahrenheit
  b. celsius
  c. avoirdupois
  d. none of the above

32. A manufacturer's bottle states that the medication be stored at controlled room temperature. The correct temperature range would be:
  a. 15-25 °C
  b. 5-10 °C
  c. 30-40 °C
  d. 0-5 °C

33. A charge which takes into account the expenses of filling a prescription is the:
  a. cost
  b. markup
  c. dispensing fee
  d. AWP

34. The compounding of non-sterile products is regulated by:
  a. CSA 345
  b. FDA 975
  c. USP 795
  d. UPS 797

35. True or False: A log book must be kept if the pharmacy repackages bulk quantities of prescription medication into unit dose packaging.
  a. true
  b. false

36. Which of the following is required when performing non-sterile compounding?
  a. well trained personnel
  b. equipment that is in good working order
  c. a suitable area intended for that purpose
  d. all of the above

37. True or False: USP 795 states that "for non-sterile solid and liquid dosage forms that are repackaged in single-unit and unit-dose containers, the beyond use date shall be one year from the date packaged or the beyond-use date on the manufacturer's container, whichever is later."
  a. true
  b. false

38. Which is the correct DAW code to use when a doctor states that a brand name product is necessary?
  a. 0

b. 1
c. 2
d. 5

39. When sending expired drugs out for destruction, a pharmacy often uses a:
    a. third party payer
    b. institutional pharmacy
    c. prescription repackager
    d. reverse distributor

40. USP 797 regulates:
    a. non-sterile compounding
    b. sterile compounding
    c. new drug approval
    d. none of the above

41. The acronym "USP" stands for:
    a. United States Pharmacies
    b. Union of Service Providers
    c. Uniform Standard Program
    d. United States Pharmacopeia

42. USP 797 covers which areas of the compounding process?
    a. equipment
    b. techniques
    c. quality control
    d. all of the above

43. The area of the pharmacy that contains the actual workspace for compounding sterile products is known as the:
    a. ante-room
    b. clean room
    c. sub station
    d. none of the above

44. The standards regarding the cleanliness of the air in the sterile compounding area is set by the:
    a. Drug Enforcement Administration
    b. Environmental Protection Agency
    c. International Organization for Standardization
    d. Profession of Aseptic Pharmacies

45. According to USP 797, the air quality inside the laminar flow hood must be:
    a. ISO Class 1
    b. ISO Class 5
    c. ISO Class 7
    d. ISO Class 8

46. Air quality testing in the clean room must be done:
    a. every six months
    b. any time we move fixtures around in the room

    c. both a & b
    d. none of the above

47. True or False: You should always put on sterile gloves before donning a sterile gown.
    a. true
    b. false

48. Periodically, throughout the workday, the work surfaces and the laminar flow hood surfaces in the clean room should be wiped with:
    a. sterile water
    b. 50% acetone
    c. 3% acetic acid
    d. 70% alcohol

49. True or False: Since you will be wearing sterile gloves, there is no reason to wash your hands before putting on your gloves.
    a. true
    b. false

50. True or False: When using proper hand washing technique, you should always position your arms in a "hands up" position until they are dry.
    a. true
    b. false

Math Test Number Three

1. Calculate the appropriate dose for an 80kg man when the recommended dose is 45mg/kg qD
      a. 1,636mg
      b. 3.6g
      c. 7,920mg
      d. 6.4g

2. What would the appropriate daily dose be for a drug given at a recommended dose of 23mg/kg TID, when the patient weighs 35kg?
      a. 404mg
      b. 805mg
      c. 1230mg
      d. 2415mg

3. A drug is to be dosed at 40mg/kg qD. What would the appropriate dose be for a 110lb female?
      a. 1.0g
      b. 2.0g
      c. 2.2g
      d. 4.4g

4. The recommended dose for Drug "A" is 30mg/kg q8h. How much of Drug "A" should be given for each dose, with a patient weighing 245lb?
      a. 2,438mg
      b. 3,341mg
      c. 7,315mg
      d. 10,022mg

5. Drug "C" is to be given at a dose of 0.3mg/kg q6h. How much should a 180lb adult be given for each dose?
      a. 12.5mg
      b. 24.5mg
      c. 45.9mg
      d. 73.6mg

6. A 2 year old child weighs 30lbs. The adult dose for Drug "C" is 250mg. Based on Young's rule, what dose should the child receive?
      a. 18mg
      b. 21mg
      c. 36mg
      d. 42mg

7. A child who weighs 18kg requires a drug who's adult dose is 120mg TID. Calculate the daily dose required using Clark's rule.
    a. 25mg
    b. 95mg
    c. 112mg
    d. 125mg

8. A patient receives 1L of IV solution over a 5 hour period. What was the flow rate in ml/hr?
    a. 125ml/hr
    b. 150ml/hr
    c. 175ml/hr
    d. 200ml/hr

9. A patient receives 750ml of IV solution over a 3 hour period. The flow rate was:
    a. 3.4ml/min
    b. 4.2ml/min
    c. 230ml/hr
    d. 280ml/hr

10. An IV of D5W is to be run for 6 hours at 75ml/hr. What volume of solution will be required?
    a. 250ml
    b. 450ml
    c. 750ml
    d. 1000ml

11. How many hours will 750ml of NS last if it is run at 80ml/hr?
    a. 3.5
    b. 6.0
    c. 7.5
    d. 9.4

12. How many liters of D5NS will be needed to run for a period of 24 hours at 125ml/hr?
    a. three
    b. seven
    c. fifteen
    d. thirty

13. 250mg of ampicillin is diluted to a final volume of 100ml. The order calls for its administration over 1 hour. Our administration set is calibrated to deliver 10gtt/ml. Calculate the appropriate rate in gtts/min.
    a. 5
    b. 8
    c. 17
    d. 24

14. 15,000 units of heparin are contained in a 500ml bag of D5W. The order calls for 750units to be given every hour. What is the correct flow rate in gtt/min? (Our administration set is calibrated at 15gtt/ml)

    a. 6
    b. 12
    c. 18
    d. 24

15. A seizure medicine is to be given at a rate of 100mg over 8 hours. The IV we have prepared contains 500mg of the drug in 1L of solution. If our administration set is calibrated to 15gtt/ml, what is the appropriate rate in gtt/min?

    a. 2
    b. 4
    c. 6
    d. 8

Section Test Number Four

1. The reference book of drug equivalence is called:
   a. the PDR
   b. the Merck Manual
   c. the orange book
   d. Fact's and Comparisons

2. The acronym DESI stands for:
   a. Drug Elimination Study Information
   b. Drug Existence Stability Information
   c. Drug Equivalence and Safety Investigation
   d. Drug Efficacy Study Implementation

3. DESI studied drugs which were:
   a. thought to be ineffective
   b. placed into use between 1938 and 1962
   c. orphan drugs
   d. not reviewed prior to 1973

4. In a bioequivalence study, a drug may be considered to be equivalent if the applicant drug's rate and extent of absorption differs from the standard drug by less than:
   a. -20%/+25%
   b. -10%/+10%
   c. -5%/+5%
   d. 0/+5%

5. If a drug has an orange book rating of "BD", it means the drug:
   a. has been proven through testing to be bioequivalent
   b. is thought to have potential bioequivalency problems
   c. has been proven through testing to not be equivalent
   d. has insufficient evidence to determine bioequivalence

6. The orange book rating of drugs which are thought to be equivalent to their standard will always start out with the letter:
   a. A
   b. B
   c. C
   c. D

7. In order to be pharmaceutical equivalents, two drugs must share all of the following, except:
   a. same drug entity
   b. same route of administration
   c. same mechanism of release
   d. same drug strength

8. Erythromycin stearate 250mg tabs and erythromycin base 250mg tabs are:
    a. pharmaceutical equivalents
    b. pharmaceutical alternatives
    c. bioequivalent
    d. therapeutic equivalents

9. The term bioavailability refers to a drug's:
    a. route of elimination
    b. half-life
    c. steady state level
    d. rate and extent of absorption

10. The organization in charge of determining a drug's bioequivalence is the:
    a. FDA
    b. DEA
    c. state board of pharmacy
    d. none of the above

11. A therapeutic equivalent drug must be both _____ and _____
    a. a pharmaceutical alternative and bioequivalent
    b. a pharmaceutical equivalent and "BD" rated
    c. a pharmaceutical equivalent and bioequivalent
    d. none of the above

12. The science of substances used to prevent, diagnose, and treat disease is:
    a. biology
    b. cosmology
    c. toxicology
    d. pharmacology

13. The spot in the body where a drug exerts its effect by controlling some sort of regulatory response is the:
    a. binder
    b. van der Waal's spot
    c. receptor
    d. none of the above

14. A drug which causes a biological process to occur is called a(n):
    a. agonist
    b. antagonist
    c. parenteral
    d. blocker

15. Potency has to do with:
    a. the number of mg contained in the product
    b. the amount of the drug required to achieve a desired result
    c. a drug's rate of absorption
    d. all of the above

16. In order to be biologically active, a drug must have all of the following properties, except:
    a. the right chemical structure and size
    b. the correct chemical bond activity
    c. bioequivalence
    d. the correct shape

17. Choose the strongest bond:
    a. covalent
    b. ionic
    c. electrostatic
    d. van der Waal's

18. When dealing with optical isomers of a drug, which isomer is usually more active?
    a. dextro-rotatory
    b. levo-rotatory
    c. a mixture of the two isomers
    d. none of the above

19. Diuretics work by:
    a. decreasing the reabsorption of sodium and potassium in the kidney
    b. decreasing the force of the heartbeat
    c. blocking angiotensin II receptors
    d. blocking calcium channels in smooth muscle

20. Given the name valsartan, this drug is most likely a(n):
    a. beta blocker
    b. calcium channel blocker
    c. ARA
    d. diuretic

21. Your patient complains of a dry hacking cough which has persisted for the last month. His profile shows he is taking the medicines listed below. Which drug may be the one which is causing the cough?
    a. HCTZ
    b. verapamil
    c. gemfibrozil
    d. captopril

22. Nasal decongestant sprays can cause a problem involving rebound congestion. How can this problem be avoided?
    a. use the medication at bedtime only
    b. take the medication with food
    c. do not use the medicine for more than 3 days straight
    d. use the drops instead of the spray

23. You just saw a patient vigorously shake her NPH insulin before use. You should tell her:
    a. wait until the bubbles are gone to use the insulin
    b. NPH insulin should not require mixing
    c. never shake insulin - gently roll it between the palms to mix
    d. none of the above

24. Accolate and Singulair are asthma medications which work by:
    a. blocking Leukotriene receptors
    b. blocking beta receptors
    c. stimulating leukotriene receptors
    d. stimulating beta receptors

25. Which of the following is false about rosiglitazone?
    a. it increases insulin release from the pancreas
    b. it increases glucose uptake in the tissues
    c. it decreases glucose production in the body
    d. it may be used with a sulfonylurea for a synergistic action

26. Which of the following is used in absence seizures?
    a. phenytoin
    b. carbamazepine
    c. gabapentin
    d. ethosuximide

27. Which should not be used in a patient with a history of seizure disorder?
    a. diazepam
    b. bupropion
    c. phenytoin
    d. atenolol

28. Which would be the most effective at lowering stomach acid levels?
    a. ranitidine
    b. nizatidine
    c. omeprazole
    d. cimetidine

29. Which of the following has the greatest risk of drug interactions?
    a. cimetidine
    b. nizatidine
    c. ranitidine
    d. famotidine

30. Which of the following is a bulk forming laxative?
    a. milk of magnesia
    b. senokot
    c. loperamide
    d. polycarbophil

31. The drug clarithromycin, is from which class of antibiotics?
    a. penicillin
    b. cephalosporin
    c. macrolide
    d. aminoglycoside

32. True or False: Blood pressure is a constant reading which rarely changes.
    a. true
    b. false

33. Diuretics exert their effects by:
    a. blocking the reabsorption of Cadmium in the kidneys
    b. blocking an enzyme in the kidneys
    c. blocking nerve message to the heart
    d. none of the above

34. Which type of diuretic is chlorthalidone?
    a. thiazide
    b. loop
    c. potassium sparring
    d. none of the above

35. Which of the following is the most potent diuretic?
    a. metolazone
    b. indapamide.
    c. hydrochlorothiazide
    d. bumetanide

36. Beta blockers which work on the heart ideally would have specificity for which receptor?
    a. beta 1
    b. beta 2
    c. beta 3
    d. beta 4

37. Which of the following classes of medication is associated with the side effect of a dry hacking cough.
    a. beta blockers
    b. ACE inhibitors
    c. ARA's
    d. calcium channel blockers

38. The drug Norvasc belongs to which category of drugs?
    a. beta blockers
    b. ACE inhibitors
    c. ARA's
    d. calcium channel blockers

39. Calcium channel blockers have effects on:
    a. vascular smooth muscle
    b. electrical impulses in the heart
    c. both a &b
    d. none of the above

40. Angina is often treated using which of these categories of medications?
    a. nitrates
    b. beta blockers
    c. calcium channel blockers
    d. all of the above

41. Digoxin is used in the treatment of:
    a. hypertension
    b. congestive heart failure
    c. hyperlipidemia
    d. blood clotting disorders

42. Which of the following drug categories would be the best choice for a patient with very high triglycerides but normal cholesterol?
    a. niacin
    b. cholestyramine
    c. fenofibrate
    d. lovastatin

43. Side effects of the HMG-CoA Reductase medications (statins) include all of the following except:
    a. liver damage
    b. muscle problems
    c. urinary retention
    d. constipation

44. Which of the following inhalers should not be used for "rescue" use of an acute asthma attack?
    a. albuterol
    b. metaproterenol
    c. levalbuterol
    d. salmeterol

45. Which of the following antihistamines would most likely cause the least sedation in a patient?
    a. chlorpheniramine
    b fexofenadine
    c. diphenhydramine
    d. carbinoxamine

46. Which of the following insulin products has the longest duration of action?
    a. NPH insulin
    b. insulin lispro
    c. insulin glargine
    d. regular insulin

47. Oral diabetes medications can work by all of the following means, except:
    a. stimulate the release of the body's own insulin
    b. inhibit the release of renin from the liver
    c. improve the body's sensitivity to insulin
    d. slow the breakdown of starches

48. Which of the following is incorrect about sulfonamide antibiotics?
    a. they can cause photosensitivity
    b. they are bactericidal
    c. they can crystallize in the urine
    d. they can cause blood problems

49. Which of the following antibiotics can cause hearing loss when given at high doses?
    a. gentamycin
    b. ciprofloxacin
    c. penicillin VK
    d. cephradine

50. Which of the following antibiotics would not be a good choice to give a marathon runner of other choices are available?
    a. gentamycin
    b. ciprofloxacin
    c. penicillin VK
    d. cephradine

Section Test Number Five

1. The process of a drug being moved from its site of administration into the blood stream is known as the drug's:
     a. absorption
     b. distribution
     c. metabolism
     d. elimination

2. Metabolism of a drug can:
     a. make an active drug inactive
     b. make an inactive drug active
     c. attach a chemical "handle" to make elimination easier
     d. all of the above

3. If a drug follows first order kinetics, and has a half-life of 2 hours, complete the following table:

TIME	BLOOD LEVEL
Start	60mg
2 hours	?
4 hours	?
6 hours	?

     a. 30,0,0
     b. 30,20,10
     c. 30,15,7.5
     d. none of the above

4. For a drug which follows first order kinetics, it takes _____ half-lives to reach steady state when repeated doses of the medication are given.
     a. 1 ½
     b. 3 ½
     c. 4 ½
     d. 7 ½

5. A drug whose metabolic pathway can be saturated, resulting in a constant rate of elimination regardless of the amount of drug given above this saturation point, is following _____ order kinetics.
     a. first
     b. zero
     c. second
     d. third

6. Invoices for controlled substances must be retained at the pharmacy for:
     a. 6 months
     b. 1 year
     c. 2 years
     d. 5 years

7. Prescriptions for controlled substances must be retained at the pharmacy until:
    a. 2 years after the date written
    b. 2 years after the last date of filling
    c. 5 years after the date written
    d. 5 years after the last date of filling

8. Schedule II and schedule III through V prescriptions:
    a. may be filed together
    b. must be filed separately from each other
    c. need to be stamped with a red "C"
    d. none of the above

9. Rent and Utilities are examples of:
    a. controllable expenses
    b. renewable expenses
    c. repeating expenses
    d. non-controllable expenses

10. An excellent place to check on the financial health of a pharmacy is the:
    a. pharmacy's checkbook
    b. accounts receivable file
    c. outstanding invoice record
    d. P&L

11. An excellent indicator of the efficient use of a pharmacy's inventory dollars is the:
    a. P&L
    b. returns record
    c. invoice register
    d. number of turns per year

12. If your pharmacy sells more than _____% of their controlled substance purchases to buyers other than the ultimate user, you must be licensed as a distributor of controlled substances.
    a. 5
    b. 10
    c. 15
    d. 20

13. Pharmacognosy is defined as:
    a. the study of how synthetic drugs affect the body
    b. the study of the side effects of drugs
    c. the study of the medicinal properties of plants and herbs
    d. the study of antibiotic activities of drugs

14. Which of the following laws pertains to natural products?
    a. DSHEA
    b. OSHA
    c. HIPAA
    d. FFDCA

15. The product Valerian may be effective in treating:
    a. diabetes
    b. insomnia
    c. prostate enlargement
    d. high blood pressure

16. Black Cohash should be used with great caution by patients who have:
    a. an allergy to aspirin
    b. diabetes
    c. an upper respiratory infection
    d. all of the above

17. A patient searching for a natural product to treat osteoarthritis of the knee would be best served by using:
    a. chamomile
    b. valerian
    c. feverfew
    d. glucosamine

18. True or False: All dietary supplements making a claim of effectiveness or purpose of use must bear the disclaimer, "This statement has not been evaluated by the Food and Drug Administration. This product is not meant to diagnose, treat, cure, or prevent any disease."
    a. true
    b. false

19. Varivax is a vaccine used to treat:
    a. flu
    b. mumps
    c. chickenpox
    d. hepatitis

20. At 9 months of age, an infant should be vaccinated with:
    a. HBV
    b. IPV
    c. both of the above
    d. none of the above

21. How often should a normal, healthy, 70 year old be vaccinated for pneumonia?
    a. every year
    b. every two years
    c. every five years
    d. every ten years

22. Which of the following needle sizes should be used to administer a vaccine via the subcutaneous route?
    a. 1 inch 18 gauge
    b. 3 inch 25 gauge
    c. ¾ inch 25 gauge
    d. ¾ inch 18 gauge

23. In an adult patient, the HBV vaccine should be administered in which location?
    a. the deltoid muscle
    b. the back of the upper arm
    c. the calf
    d. the bicep

24. A complete inventory of your controlled substances must be done at least every:
    a. 6 months
    b. 12 months
    c. two years
    d. five years

25. In addition to the count of controlled substances, the biennial inventory record must include which of the following?
    a. the name of the people conducting the inventory
    b. the name and address of the pharmacy
    c. whether it was done before opening or after closing on that date
    d. all of the above

26. During a biennial controlled substance inventory, for bottles less than 1,000 dosage units you should count by:
    a. individual doses (ie, 175 units)
    b. number of full and partial bottles (ie, 1.75 bottles)
    c. ignoring any packages of less than 1,000 doses
    d. none of the above

27. True or False: the biennial inventory is another name for the perpetual inventory.
    a. true
    b. false

28. Which of the following statements about OSHA is incorrect?
    a. it is a division of the U.S. Department of Labor
    b. it affects only employers with over 500 employees
    c. it's mission statement includes saving lives, preventing injuries, and protecting the health of workers
    d. it was put into law by Congress in 1970

29. Under OSHA regulations, employers must do all of the following, except:
    a. provide a safe place to work
    b. make safety equipment available for those who choose to use it
    c. keep adequate records of occupational accidents
    d. correct recognizable hazards

30. If a violation occurs, OSHA has the ability to assess:
    a. a fine
    b. a citation
    c. jail time
    d. all of the above

31. True or False: An employer should have a binder containing the MSDS for all chemicals used in your local area of town.
    a. true
    b. false

32. What is the purpose of the MSDS for a product?
    a. to obtain information on hazardous materials in the workplace
    b. to obtain the average wholesale cost of a product
    c. to record materials received by the pharmacy
    d. to record how often a product is used in the pharmacy

33. True or False: If you need to find out if a product contains hazardous material, you should check its MSDS sheet.
    a. true
    b. false

34. True or False: Most hazardous waste found in a pharmacy can safely be disposed of down the sink drain.
    a. true
    b. false

35. Which of the following products is considered a hazardous waste when it can no longer be dispensed?
    a. atenolol
    b. lisinopril
    c. penicillin
    d. warfarin

36. True or False: Hazardous waste must be picked up by a licensed hazardous waste company for destruction.
    a. true
    b. false

37. Whenever a spill of a product occurs in the pharmacy you should:
    a. check the products MSDS for clean up instructions
    b. wear PPE for any hazardous or caustic chemicals
    c. warn coworkers and customers in the area of the spill
    d. all of the above

38. General housekeeping in the pharmacy includes all of the following, except:
    a. keeping floors clean and dry
    b. keeping the isles free of trip hazards
    c. keeping exit doors locked and unblocked
    d. keeping flammable products stored properly

39. Medication errors can include which of the following?
    a. prescribing errors
    b. dispensing errors
    c. patient adherence issues
    d. all of the above

40. It is estimated that dispensing errors account for up to _____% of all medication errors in the retail pharmacy environment.
    a. 12.5%
    b. 24%
    c. 66%
    d. 95%

41. The failure to give a dose of medication to a hospital patient would be considered what type of medication error?
    a. prescribing error
    b. omission error
    c. wrong dose error
    d. dispensing error

42. If in the process of filling a prescription we find that a drug that should have been in the refrigerator was on our regular pharmacy shelves for a prolonged period of time. If we were to use that product in filling the prescription we could be creating a medication error of the following type:
    a. adherence error
    b. storage error
    c. deteriorated drug error
    d. dispensing error

43. It has been estimated that 25% of all dispensing errors in the past were caused by:
    a. prescriber handwriting
    b. wrong drug strength
    c. wrong patient name
    d. distractions in the pharmacy

44. Which of the following is not a common cause of medication errors?
    a. illegible prescriptions
    b. look-alike drug names
    c. inappropriate writing of decimal strengths
    d. well trained pharmacy personnel

45. Which of the following factors have contributed to a decrease in medication errors in the pharmacy?
    a. use of bar codes
    b. organization in the pharmacy
    c. electronic prescribing
    d. all of the above

46. True or False: TQM efforts concentrate on the quality of outcomes and the processes involved, rather than on individual mistakes
    a. true
    b. false

47. A good TQM program will include all of the following, except:
    a. logging pharmacy events in a notebook
    b. frequent TQM meetings for just the pharmacists involved
    c. a plan of action to help prevent future events
    d. maintaining a record of the TQM meeting and discarding the event logs

48. True or False: One of the best ways to eliminate look-alike and sound-alike product confusion is to group them together on one spot on the pharmacy shelves.
    a. true
    b. false

49. It is estimated that by using proper patient counseling techniques, approximately _____% of medication errors can be caught.
    a. 25%
    b. 55%
    c. 83%
    d. 96%

50. Patient counseling is important because:
    a. it helps the patient use their drugs correctly
    b. it helps eliminate drug errors reaching the patient
    c. both of the above
    d. none of the above

Final Examination #1

1. The maximum number of refills that an alprazolam prescription can have is:
    a. 5
    b. 12
    c. an unlimited number within one year
    d. no refills are allowed

2. A 1% Triamcinolone cream is ordered for a hospital patient. The manner in which this drug will be dispensed is most likely:
    a. unit dose
    b. bulk drug
    c. prn drug
    d. floor stock

3. The use of a locking cap for prescription vials was mandated by the:
    a. SETI
    b. OBRA
    c. PPPA
    d. CIA

4. You are typing a label for a prescription which reads: 1-2gtts OD TID prn. The label should read:
    a. Instill 1 or 2 drops in the left ear 3 times daily as needed
    b. Instill 1 or 2 drops in the right ear 3 times daily as needed
    c. Instill 1 or 2 drops in the right eye 3 times daily as needed
    d. Instill 1 or 2 drops in the left eye 3 times daily as needed

5. Which area of the pharmacy would contain the laminar flow hood?
    a. the ante room
    b. the clean room
    c. the nursing station
    d. the out patient pharmacy

6. Our package states to, "Store at 0 °C to 5 °C". Where should we keep the product?
    a. room temperature
    b. in the refrigerator
    c. in the freezer
    d. in un-reconstituted powder form only

7. A brand name of Verapamil is:
    a. Calan
    b. Hytrin
    c. Norvasc
    d. Aldomet

8. The generic name for Lopressor is:
   a. atenolol
   b. acebutolol
   c. metoprolol
   d. sotalol

9. Given the name lisinopril, this drug is most likely a:
   a. diuretic
   b. ACE inhibitor
   c. beta blocker
   d. calcium channel blocker

10. A major concern while using venlafaxine on a patient is the drug's ability to:
    a. slow the heartbeat
    b. cause irreversible liver damage
    c. cause hypoglycemia
    d. increase blood pressure

11. Dr. Jones has a hypertensive patient for whom he will be prescribing a blood pressure medication. Dr. Jones knows he should not prescribe a non-specific beta blocker for this patient. The patient is most likely:
    a. pregnant
    b. an asthmatic
    c. obese
    d. an epileptic

12. Earlier in the day, Dr. Jones saw a 6 year old patient who has an infection. The antibiotic class he should have avoided prescribing for this patient is:
    a. penicillins
    b. tetracyclines
    c. cephalosporins
    d. sulfonamides

13. The pharmacy's torsion balance should not be used to weigh amounts less than:
    a. 100 gm
    b. 100 mg
    c. 60 mg
    d. 6 mg

14. A meniscus is a phenomenon which occurs when:
    a. a cream is mixed with an emulsion
    b. a liquid is measured in a glass cylinder
    c. a needle is not tilted when it punctures and passes through a rubber stopper
    d. an error is discovered in the pharmacy

15. Which of the following is not a reference you would expect to see in the pharmacy?
    a. Facts & Comparisons
    b. MSDS
    c. Pharmacy Practice Act
    d. ASPCA book

16. The primary organ used in drug metabolism is the:
    a. stomach
    b. liver
    c. intestine
    d. kidney

17. Before an oral drug can get into the systemic circulation, it passes through the:
    a. pancreas
    b. liver
    c. kidneys
    d. heart

18. A product rated "AT" in the orange book would be considered to be:
    a. bioequivalent
    b. not bioequivalent

19. A doctor writes the following prescription: Bactrim Suspension 2 tsp po BID x 10d
    How many total milliliters does the patient receive each day?
    a. 5
    b. 10
    c. 15
    d. 20

20. In the above problem, what would be the total number of milliliters needed to complete the therapy?
    a. 100
    b. 200
    c. 150
    d. 175

21. The cost of atenolol 50mg is $5.88 per 100 tabs. What is the cost for 58 tablets?
    a. $3.41
    b. $2.88
    c. $0.87
    d. $5.63

22. In the NDC number 00034-4536-13, the digits 4536 indicate:
    a. the expiration date of the drug
    b. the package size of the drug
    c. the manufacturer of the drug
    d. the drug contained in the package

23. The process in which a drug enters the body is called:
    a. absorption
    b. distribution
    c. metabolism
    d. elimination

24. The process of absorption, distribution, and elimination of a drug from the body constitutes a drug's _____ profile
    a. equivalence
    b. pharmacokinetic
    c. toxicological
    d. therapeutic

25. Which of the following will not be found on an MAR?
    a. the prescriber's name
    b. the patient's location
    c. a list of concurrent medications
    d. the dosing schedule

26. What is the chemical formula for normal saline?
    a. NaCl
    b. KCl
    c. MgSO4
    d. Na+

27. Determine the correct selling price of a drug which costs us $9.89, if we have a 58% markup and a $2.00 dispensing fee.
    a. $17.63
    b. $23.88
    c. $37.28
    d. $10.99

28. Which of the following drug recall levels should pharmacy personnel be most concerned with?
    a. class I
    b. class II
    c. class III
    d. class IV

29. The agency which would have issued the above recall is the:
    a. FDA
    b. DEA
    c. OSHA
    d. AMA

30. The classification which may not have refills is:
    a. schedule II
    b. schedule III
    c. schedule IV
    d. schedule V

31. True or False: 1 lb. is equal to 2.2 kg.
    a. true
    b. false

32. A prescription calls for 1000ml of 30% Dextrose. Your pharmacy stocks Dextrose as a 70% solution. How much sterile water should you mix with 70% Dextrose to get the final product?
    a. 375 ml
    b. 571 ml
    c. 125 ml
    d. 288 ml

33. 47. How many tablets should be dispensed to fill the following prescription? Prednisone 5mg tabs - 30mg qD x 3d, then 20mg qD x 3d, then 10mg qD x 3d, then 5mg qD x 10d
    a. 12
    b. 19
    c. 39
    d. 46

34. The first letter in a physician's assistant DEA number will be:
    a. an "M"
    b. the first letter in the doctor's last name
    c. an "A" or "B"
    d. any letter assigned by the DEA

35. A pharmacy technician can perform all of the following except:
    a. bulk compounding
    b. ask a patient about their drug allergies
    c. process a patient's third party information
    d. accept a new telephoned prescription from a doctor

36. In accepting a prescription written for diazepam, you note that the patient wants brand name only. The correct medicine to use would be:
    a. Klonopin
    b. Xanax
    c. Dyazide
    d. Valium

37. When reviewing a patient's profile, you notice that their new prescription for chlordiazepoxide may be a duplication with another one they already have. Which of the following would cause a drug duplication with today's prescription?
    a. HCTZ 50mg po qam
    b. atenolol 50mg po qD
    c. Calan SR 240mg po qD
    d. alprazolam 0.05mg TID prn

38. A prescription calls for 3oz of Hydrocortisone cream. The correct amount to dispense is:
    a. 15g
    b. 30g
    c. 60g
    d. 90g

39. The HIPAA law primarily concerns itself with:
    a. patient privacy
    b. drug safety
    c. drug stability
    d. drug purity

40. Which of the following legislation was an attempt to curb importation of unsafe drugs from other countries?
    a. The Durham-Humphrey Amendment
    b. The Federal Food, Drug, and Cosmetic Act
    c. The Prescription Drug Marketing Act
    d. The FDA Modernization Act

41. The major source of contamination when working in the laminar flow hood is:
    a. the syringe
    b. the IV bag
    c. the medicine vial
    d. the person working in the hood

42. An IV bag is to run at 500ml over 8 hours. Our administrated set is calibrated at 15gtt/ml. Calculate the appropriate flow rate in gtts/min.
    a. 10
    b. 12
    c. 16
    d. 20

43. If 42g of a product occupies 30ml of volume, how many ml will 89g occupy?
    a. 64
    b. 48
    c. 120
    d. 88

44. Which of the following drugs should never be stopped abruptly?
    a. leukotriene modifiers
    b. diuretics
    c. clonidine
    d. antihistamines

45. ACE inhibitors cause their antihypertensive effect by:
    a. blocking angiotensin II receptors
    b. inhibiting the conversion of angiotensin I to angiotensin II
    c. blocking receptors at the heart
    d. causing diuresis

46. Acetaminophen (APAP) is dosed at 10mg/kg q6h. Our patient weighs 38lb. The APAP we will use is a solution containing 80mg per ½ teaspoonful. What would be the correct amount to give the patient for each dose?
    a. 5.4ml
    b. 2.7ml
    c. 10.6ml
    d. 3.4ml

47. 256oz is equal to how many liters?
    a. 7.68
    b. 7680
    c. 2.56
    d. 2560

48. A chemical spill has just occurred in the pharmacy. What reference would be the best source of information regarding the safe cleanup of the product?
    a. orange book
    b. Facts & Comparisons
    c. US Pharmacopea
    d. MSDS book

49. Which DEA schedule contains drugs with no current acceptable medical use?
    a. Schedule IV
    b. Schedule III
    c. Schedule II
    d. Schedule I

50. You have received a new IV pump from the manufacturer. Your institution's protocol states that you must verify the calibration of the unit before you can put it into general use. The label on the unit says it will deliver 15gtt/ml. You test run 50ml of solution through the pump, which takes exactly 30 minutes to run. The count you made showed that there were 25gtts delivered by the machine every minute. Should this unit now be used on patients?
    a. yes, the results are exactly what was expected based on the unit's stated calibration
    b. no, the unit delivered too many gtt/ml
    c. no, the unit delivered too few gtt/ml
    d. there is not enough information to determine the accuracy of the pump

51. Dr. Jones wants to give insulin to his patient to get an immediate decrease in his dangerously high blood glucose levels. He wants to know which type of insulin your pharmacist would recommend. Based on your knowledge of insulin products, which would be the appropriate recommendation for the pharmacist to make?
    a. Humulin R
    b. Humulin N
    c. Levemir
    d. Lantus

52. We have a hospital patient who is a 30lb 4 y/o male. The doctor wants to give an injection of Drug "A" to the patient. The package insert for "A" states that the adult dose is 250mg. There is no pediatric dosing specified. Using Young's rule, calculate the appropriate dose for the child.
    a. 41.67 mg
    b. 62.5mg
    c. 83.8 mg
    d. 94.7 mg

53. How much hydrocortisone would be present in 300g of a 2.5% cream?
    a. 3 g
    b. 4.5 g
    c. 7.5 g
    d. 25 g

54. Pseudomembranous colitis is a possible side effect of which group of medication?
    a. antibiotics
    b. beta blockers
    c. diuretics
    d. H2 antagonists

55. Which group of antibiotics works by weakening the cell wall of the reproducing bacteria?
    a. macrolides
    b. flouroquinolones
    c. tetracyclines
    d. penicillins

56. A patient who has had an allergic reaction to Dynabac would most likely be cross sensitive to:
    a. erythromycin
    b. gentamycin
    c. ciprofloxacin
    d. tetracycline

57. Which of the following is a stimulant laxative?
    a. MOM
    b. polycarbophil
    c. bisacodyl
    d. loperamide

58. Which of the following is a proton pump inhibitor?
    a. nizatidine
    b. ompeprazole
    c. cisapride
    d. gatifloxacin

59. All of the following would need to appear on the unit dose packaging of a medication, except:
    a. the name of the drug
    b. the expiration date
    c. the lot number
    d. the patient's name

60. Which of the following is true about Phenytoin?
    a. it is relatively free of drug interaction potential
    b. it may be discontinued without a taper down period
    c. it has a wide therapeutic range
    d. the patient should notify their dentist that they are on the medication

61. Pharmacy technicians can perform their duties provided they:
    a. are certified
    b. double check everything they do
    c. work only under assigned protocols
    d. have all labels and products checked by a pharmacist

62. The correct abbreviation for "left eye" is:
    a. OS
    b. OD
    c. AS
    d. AD

63. Which DEA schedule contains products which may be dispensed by a pharmacist without a prescription?
    a. all controlled substances require a prescription before they can be sold
    b. schedule III
    c. schedule IV
    d. schedule V

64. A major concern with topical decongestant products is:
    a. they may cause an increase in ocular pressure with glaucoma patients
    b. they may cause rebound congestion
    c. they are teratogenic
    d. they may cause first dose syncope

65. Which site of injection will give the fastest rate of absorption for SQ insulin?
    a. arm
    b. thigh
    c. abdomen
    d. all are the same

66. The term "transdermal" indicates drug delivery through:
    a. injection
    b. oral use
    c. topical use
    d. none of the above

67. If the FDA is going to issue a recall for a medication which will cause serious health consequences or death as a result of use, which class recall will it be?
    a. I
    b. II
    c. III
    d. IV

68. Which of the following classes of antibiotics show a cross sensitivity with penicillin?
    a. macrolide
    b. flouroquinolone
    c. cephalosporin
    d. aminoglycoside

69. When more than one law would apply in a given situation, which law would apply?
   a. the state law
   b. the federal law
   c. the DEA law
   d. the most stringent law would apply

70. The form on which schedule II drugs are ordered is called the:
   a. DEA 921 form
   b. DEA 222 form
   c. FDA 921 form
   d. FDA 222 form

71. The formula most often used for reimbursement under third party contracts states:
   _____ ± % + dispensing fee = selling price
   a. cost
   b. expenses
   c. AWP
   d. none of the above

72. An invoice for Vicodin received at the pharmacy must be retained for:
   a. 2 years
   b. 1 year
   c. 6 months
   d. there is no requirement to keep it

73. A laminar flow HEPA filter should be professionally checked every:
   a. month
   b. 3 months
   c. 6 months
   d. 1 year

74. Who is responsible for approving new drug entities?
   a. the Drug Enforcement Administration
   b. the State Board of Pharmacy
   c. the Pharmacy Practice Act
   d. the Food and Drug Administration

75. A 2% solution of NaCl would be:
   a. hypertonic
   b. hypotonic
   c. isotonic
   d. none of the above

76. An enteric coated tablet should not be taken with:
   a. antacids
   b. grapefruit juice
   c. soda drinks
   d. none of the above

77. True or False: Once the designation of CPhT is earned through examination, it may be used forever without additional requirements.
   a. true
   b. false

78. The Combat Methamphetamine Act concerns itself with:
    a. Scheduled Listed Chemical Products (SLCP)
    b. Selective Serotonin Reuptake Inhibitors (SSRI)
    c. Selective Beta Blocker Antagonists (SBBA)
    d. none of the above

79. Which of the following pregnancy categories should never be used in pregnant females?
    a. A
    b. C
    c. X
    d. Z

80. Some of the more important provisions of the HITECH legislation include all of the following, except:
    a. gives online PHI access to the patient
    b. strengthens the electronic security of PHI
    c. clarifies who may access a patient's PHI
    d. eliminates the need for notice of breaches of PHI

81. Which of the following may be an indication that a prescription might be forged?
    a. the prescription looks "too neat"
    b. directions that vary significantly from the norm
    c. erasures or changes in the prescription
    d. all of the above

82. The main components to the e-prescribe system for prescriptions includes all of the following, except:
    a. the prescriber
    b. the transaction hub
    c. the patient's PBM if they are on insurance
    d. the state police clearing house

83. True or False: According to federal law, a prescription for a Schedule II controlled substance may be transmitted electronically if the prescriber and pharmacy have the required software.
    a. true
    b. false

84. When measuring a volume of liquid in a syringe, you should always take your reading using the:
    a. black ring of the plunger closest to the tip
    b. black ting of the plunger furthest from the tip
    c. end of the plunger
    d. none of the above

85. Which of the following is a class of medications that require the distribution of an FDA approved Medication Guide?
    a. loop diuretics
    b. estrogen hormones
    c. ACE inhibitors
    d. stimulant laxatives

86. What is the correct sequence for the normal hospital drug distribution process?
    a. prescriber -> pharmacist -> patient administration
    b. pharmacist -> prescriber -> patient administration
    c. prescriber -> patient administration -> pharmacist
    d. pharmacist -> prescriber -> patient administration

87. True or False: Schedule II drugs must always be ordered using a paper DEA Form 222.
    a. true
    b. false

88. The requirements of USP <797> affect:
    a. sterile compounding
    b. non-sterile compounding
    c. ordering of controlled substances
    d. approval of new drugs

89. The ante room of a sterile product compounding area must meet which ISO standard at a minimum?
    a. Class 5
    b. Class 7
    c. Class 8
    d. Class 10

90. Which of the following natural products might be useful in treating high cholesterol?
    a. garlic
    b. feverfew
    c. echinacea
    d. ginger

Final Examination #2

1. The maximum length of time an atenolol prescription may be filled is:
   a. 6 months
   b. 1 year
   c. no refills are allowed

2. What term best describes a product of oil droplets suspended in water, where the drug is usually dissolved in the oil?
   a. extract
   b. tincture
   c. emulsion
   d. semi-solid

3. Which of the following is recorded on an MAR?
   a. the mediation name
   b. the time and date a dose of the medication was given
   c. the name of the person administering the dose
   d. all of the above

4. The legislation that covers food supplements is called:
   a. SETI
   b. OBRA
   c. DSHEA
   d. CIA

5. You are typing a label for a prescription which reads: 1-2gtts AD QID prn pain. The label should read:
   a. Instill 1 or 2 drops in the left ear 4 times daily as needed for pain
   b. Instill 1 or 2 drops in the right ear 4 times daily as needed for pain
   c. Instill 1 or 2 drops in the right eye 4 times daily as needed for pain
   d. Instill 1 or 2 drops in the left eye 4 times daily as needed for pain

6. Which of the following should be utilized when preparing an injectable chemotherapy drug?
   a. a horizontal laminar flow hood
   b. a vertical laminar flow hood
   c. a random laminar flow hood
   d. technicians should never work on chemotherapy drugs

7. Our package states to, "Store at 25 °C". Where should we keep the product?
   a. room temperature
   b. in the refrigerator
   c. in the freezer
   d. in un-reconstituted powder form only

8. A complete inventory of all the pharmacy's controlled drugs must be completed every:
   a. 6 months
   b. 12 months
   c. 24 months
   d. 60 months

9. The brand name of prazosin is:
   a. Norvasc
   b. Tenormin
   c. Minipress
   d. Flexeril

10. The generic name for Tenormin is:
    a. atenolol
    b. acebutolol
    c. metoprolol
    d. sotalol

11. Given the name propranolol, this drug is most likely a:
    a. diuretic
    b. ACE inhibitor
    c. beta blocker
    d. calcium channel blocker

12. A major concern while using a diuretic on a patient is the drug's ability to:
    a. slow the heartbeat
    b. cause irreversible liver damage
    c. cause hypoglycemia
    d. cause potassium loss from the body

13. Dr. Jones has a hypertensive patient for whom he will be prescribing a blood pressure medication. Dr. Jones knows he should not prescribe Zestril for this patient. The patient is most likely:
    a. pregnant
    b. an asthmatic
    c. obese
    d. an epileptic

14. Earlier in the day, Dr. Jones saw a patient who was a type I diabetic. The hypertension medicine he should have avoided prescribing for this patient is:
    a. enalapril
    b. propranolol
    c. verapamil
    d. HCTZ

15. Tomorrow, Dr. Jones will see a patient whose chief complaint is a persistent dry cough which he's had for the last "couple of months", since he started his new blood pressure medicine. When reviewing the patient's chart you see he is taking the following medications. Which one is most likely the cause of the patient's cough?
    a. HCTZ
    b. atenolol
    c. fosinopril
    d. prazosin

16. When determining if a drug is a bioequivalent product, the proper reference book to use is the:
    a. Facts & Comparisons
    b. MSDS
    c. orange book
    d. OBRA book

17. The primary organ involved in drug elimination is the:
    a. stomach
    b. liver
    c. intestine
    d. kidney

18. The organ where respiration takes place is called the:
    a. pancreas
    b. lungs
    c. kidneys
    d. heart

19. A product rated "BB" in the orange book would be considered to be:
    a. bioequivalent
    b. not bioequivalent

20. A doctor writes the following prescription: Augmentin 400mg/5ml 7.5ml po BID x 10d How many total teaspoonfuls does the patient receive each day?
    a. 3
    b. 2
    c. 5
    d. 1

21. In the above problem, what would be the total number of milliliters needed to complete the therapy?
    a. 100
    b. 200
    c. 150
    d. 175

22. The cost of allopurinol 300mg is $39.99 per 100 tabs. What is the cost for 58 tablets?
    a. $23.19
    b. $145.04
    c. $19.89
    d. $45.98

23. Which of the following drugs is available in a topical patch formulation?
    a. prazosin
    b. enalapril
    c. clonidine
    d. losartan

24. In the NDC number 00034-4536-13, the digits 00034 indicate:
    a. the expiration date of the drug
    b. the package size of the drug
    c. the manufacturer of the drug
    d. the drug contained in the package

25. Which of the following does not need to be typed on the label of a retail prescription?
    a. the prescription number
    b. the patient's name
    c. the sig
    d. the patient's account number

26. The process which prepares a drug for removal from the body is called:
    a. absorption
    b. distribution
    c. metabolism
    d. elimination

27. The main drug packaging in the hospital is known as:
    a. prescription bottle
    b. drug envelope
    c. unit dose
    d. none of the above

28. What is the concentration of normal saline?
    a. 0.9%
    b. 1.8%
    c. 5%
    d. 10%

29. Which dosage form would best mask the unpleasant taste of a drug?
    a. a chewable tablet
    b. a buccal tablet
    c. an SL tablet
    d. a gelatin capsule

30. The main agency issues drug recall notices is the:
    a. FDA
    b. DEA
    c. OSHA
    d. AMA

31. The classification which contains drugs with the highest potential for abuse is:
    a. schedule V
    b. schedule IV
    c. schedule III
    d. schedule II

32. 1 pound is equal to:
    a. 2.2 kg
    b. 1000 mg
    c. 454 g
    d. 1000 ml

33. How much white petrolatum must be added to 20% ichthamol ointment to make 400 grams of 4% ichthamol ointment??
    a. 80 g
    b. 160 g
    c. 230 g
    d. 320 g

34. Licensing and professional regulation of pharmacies is done by the:
    a. Food and Drug Administration
    b. Drug Enforcement Administration
    c. State Board of Pharmacy
    d. United States Pharmacopea

35. The first letter in an medical doctor's DEA number will most likely be:
    a. an "A", "B", or an "F"
    b. the first letter in the doctor's last name
    c. a "V" if they are a veterinarian
    d. any letter assigned by the DEA

36. In accepting a prescription written for atorvastatin, you note that the patient wants brand name only. The correct medicine to use would be:
    a. Lipitor
    b. Vermox
    c. Valium
    d. Zocor

37. When reviewing a patient's profile, you notice that their new prescription for Tenormin may be a duplication with another one they already have. Which of the following would cause a drug duplication with today's prescription?
    a. furosemide
    b. lisinopril
    c. propranolol
    d. ranitidine

38. A prescription calls for 8oz of lactulose. The correct amount to dispense is:
    a. 30 ml
    b. 120 ml
    c. 240 ml
    d. 473 ml

39. The Federal Food and Drug Act primarily concerns itself with:
    a. patient privacy
    b. drug safety
    c. drug stability
    d. drug purity

40. Which of the following is not a cause of medication errors identified by the Institute for Safe Medication Practices?
    a. look alike drug names
    b. misunderstood abbreviations
    c. miscommunication between health care providers
    d. complete patient record keeping

41. An IV bag is to run at 500ml over 8 hours. Our administrated set is calibrated at 15gtt/ml. Calculate the appropriate flow rate in gtts/min.
    a. 10
    b. 12
    c. 16
    d. 20

42. If 500 penicillin tablets cost $39.95, how much would 800 cost us?
    a. $48.57
    b. $63.92
    c. $119.55
    d. $36.97

43. The risk of permanent ototoxicity with overdose occurs with which of the following groups of medicine?
    a. beta blockers
    b. alpha blockers
    c. thiazide diuretics
    d. loop diuretics

44. Which of the following drugs should never be stopped abruptly?
    a. beta blockers
    b. diuretics
    c. antihistamines
    d. ACE inhibitors

45. The dose of Amoxil for the infection our patient has is 40mg/kg/day in 2 divided doses. Our patient weighs 140lbs. Each dose given should be:
    a. 2,545mg
    b. 1,273mg
    c. 1,875mg
    d. 6,160mg

46. The compounding of a prescription medication for a single patient without a written protocol on file is called _____ compounding.
    a. bulk
    b. extemporaneous
    c. aseptic
    d. illegal

47. A chemical spill has just occurred in the pharmacy. What reference would be the best source of information regarding the safe cleanup of the product?
    a. orange book
    b. Facts & Comparisons
    c. US Pharmacopea
    d. MSDS book

48. Which of the following made patient counseling mandatory for all Medicaid patients?
    a. OBRA
    b. PPPA
    c. Durham-Humphrey
    d. LPGA

49. A sulfonylurea is a drug which is very similar to the sulfonamide antibiotics, yet they have no antibacterial activity themselves. What disease state is the sulfonylureas used to treat?
    a. diabetes
    b. HTN
    c. seizures
    d. depression

50. Which is correct regarding insulin?
    a. NPH should always be a clear solution
    b. it is stable for no more than 10 days at room temperature
    c. it is absorbed at the same rate regardless of injection site
    d. care must be taken never to shake or drop insulin

51. Once a drug has passed its beyond use date it is not to be used. Which of the following also becomes toxic as it ages past its beyond use date?
    a. penicillin
    b. erythromycin
    c. ciprofloxacin
    d. tetracycline

52. How many mg of KMnO4 are present in 35ml of a 1:100 solution?
    a. 3.5 mg
    b. 35 mg
    c. 350 mg
    d. 3500 mg

53. Which of the following antibiotics would pose the greatest danger to a pregnant woman and her fetus?
    a. amoxicillin
    b. cephalexin
    c. ampicillin
    d. tetracycline

54. A patient who has had an allergic reaction to Amoxil would most likely be cross sensitive to:
    a. penicillin VK
    b. gentamycin
    c. ciprofloxacin
    d. tetracycline

55. Which of the following antibiotics will interact with dairy products?
    a. amoxicillin
    b. tetracycline
    c. tobramycin
    d. dirithromycin

56. Which of the following is a bulk forming laxative?
    a. MOM
    b. polycarbophil
    c. bisacodyl
    d. loperamide

57. Which of the following is incorrect about laxatives?
    a. they should not be used for longer than 7 days
    b. fleet's phospho soda is a saline laxative
    c. laxatives are contraindicated for patients with nausea, abdominal pain, or vomitting
    d. bisacodyl is available as an oral, disintegrating, tablet

58. Which of the following influences the duties which a technician can perform?
    a. state laws
    b. pharmacist beliefs
    c. the technician's abilities
    d. all of the above

59. Which of the following drugs could not be placed back into the pharmacy inventory if they are returned?
    a. an unopened unit dose package of medication from the previous day's cart exchange
    b. a retail prescription for a non-controlled liquid in a 4oz amber oval
    c. a tube of ointment dispensed as a bulk drug which is returned with its seal intact
    d. none of the above may be reused

60. How many 30mg KMnO4 tablets would be needed to make 1.2L of a 1:1000 solution?
    a. 4
    b. 10
    c. 40
    d. 100

61. If the manufacturer's expiration date reads "12/15", the last day this product may be used is:
    a. November 30, 2015
    b. November 1, 2015
    c. December 1, 2015
    d. December 31, 2015

62. The correct abbreviation for "left ear" is:
    a. OS
    b. OD
    c. AS
    d. AD

63. Ranitidine is a histamine blocker used to treat:
    a. allergies
    b. rash
    c. excess stomach acid
    d. nervousness

64. Which of the following gauges would represent the thinnest needle?
    a. 21
    b. 18
    c. 29
    d. 23

65. All of the following would be considered a parenteral route, except:
    a. IV
    b. IM
    c. SQ
    d. NG

66. The abbreviation "D5NS" stands for:
    a. 5% Dextrose & Sterile Water
    b. 5% Dextrose & 0.45% NaCl
    c. 5% Dextrose & 0.9% NaCl
    d. 5% Dextrose & 0.9% KCl

67. Which of the following drugs is available in both prescription and OTC strengths?
    a. atenolol
    b. lisinopril
    c. famotidine
    d. oxycodone

68. Which of the following is an SSRI?
    a. sertraline
    b. doxepin
    c. amitriptyline
    d. lithium

69. Proper technique when working in the laminar flow hood is know as:
    a. aseptic technique
    b. clean room technique
    c. laminar technique
    d. vertical technique

70. You need to measure 78ml of liquid. The proper size graduated cylinder to use is:
    a. 1 oz
    b. 2 oz
    c. 3 oz
    d. 4 oz

71. The abbreviation "CHF" stands for:
    a. congestive heart failure
    b. chart home foods
    c. can have food
    d. congestion of head & fever

72. A phase I NDA trial is conducted to test a new drug's:
    a. efficacy
    b. maximum tolerated dose
    c. marketability
    d. effectiveness versus a known drug product

73. Which of the following is not a pharmacy technician certification (CPhT) organization?
    a. National Association of Boards of Pharmacy
    b. Pharmacy Technician Certification Board
    c. National Healthcare Association
    d. all of the above certify technicians (CPhT)

74. The CMEA requirements include all of the following, except:
    a. SLCP's must be kept behind the pharmacy counter
    b. a log must be kept of all sales for at least two years after the last sale
    c. all employees involved in the sale of SLCP's must have specialized training
    d. an unlimited amount of SCLP's may be purchased as long as the customer has proper identification

75. The HITECH legislation established which of the following?
    a. a maximum penalty of $250,000 for each violation
    b. strengthened security of patient PHI
    c. an easier way to approve new drug products
    d. all of the above

76. Possible reasons to contact a prescriber before filling a prescription include:
    a. drug-drug interactions
    b. possible overdose situations
    c. illegible handwriting on the prescription
    d. all of the above

77. Reasons to have a formulary in your pharmacy include:
    a. reduce drug duplication
    b. reduce treatment cost
    c. reduce inventory costs
    d. all of the above

78. Some oral antibiotics for suspension are manufactured as _____ due to their
    _____.
    a. capsules, poor taste
    b. dehydrated powders, instability in water environments
    c. syrups, great bioavailability
    d. emulsions, inherent stability

79. During the transmission of a prescription using the e-prescribe system, the link
    between the prescriber and the pharmacy is known as the:
    a. transaction hub
    b. prescription modulator
    c. checkfree system
    d. software vendor

80. True or False: According to federal law, a prescription for a Schedule IV controlled
    substance may be transmitted electronically if the prescriber and pharmacy have
    the required software.
    a. true
    b. false

81. Which of the following will cause the phenomenon known as a meniscus?
    a. liquid measured in a plastic graduated cylinder
    b. liquid measured in a glass graduated cylinder
    c. solids weighed on a torsion balance
    d. none of the above

82. Which of the following is not a reason the FDA may mandate the use of a
    Medication Guide?
    a. certain information is necessary to prevent serious side effects
    b. patient decision making should be made with information about a known
       serious side effect
    c. patient adherence to directions is critical to the drug's effectiveness
    d. the cost of a prescription is abnormally high

83. When using a paper DEA Form 222 to return expired controlled drugs to a
    reverse distributor, which copy of the 222 should you return in the box with the
    returned drugs?
    a. brown copy 1
    b. green copy 2
    c. blue copy 3
    d. none of the above

84. The advantage of the CSOS system is:
    a. greater protection of the patient PHI
    b. allows online ordering of controlled substances
    c. greater protection of the sterility of a product
    d. better inventory control in the pharmacy

85. Which of the following reconstituted antibiotic preparations should not be stored in the refrigerator?
    a. penicillin VK
    b. amoxicillin/clavulanate
    c. clarithromycin
    d. all reconstituted products require refrigeration

86. Which is the proper method for hand washing before working in a sterile environment?
    a. Wash from the elbow to the hand using a straight motion
    b. Wash from the elbow to the hand using a circular motion
    c. Wash from the hand to the elbow using a straight motion
    d. Wash from the hand to the elbow using a circular motion

87. Which of the following natural products might be useful in treating hypertension?
    a. coenzyme Q10
    b. black cohash
    c. chondroitin sulfate
    d. acidophilus

88. A vaccine that utilizes a scratch of the skin for administration is used to prevent:
    a. measles
    b. small pox
    c. pneumonia
    d. influenza

89. A "TQM" system is used to:
    a. keep PHI private
    b. return expired drugs
    c. help prevent future pharmacy errors
    d. process third party payments

90. True or False: Only the pharmacist is responsible for preventing and reducing errors made in the pharmacy.
    a. true
    b. false

Math Test Answers

Test One	Test Two	Test Three
1. c	1. a	1. b
2. c	2. c	2. d
3. b	3. a	3. b
4. a	4. c	4. b
5. d	5. b	5. b
6. a	6. d	6. c
7. c	7. b	7. b
8. a	8. a	8. d
9. a	9. c	9 b
10. c	10. a	10. b
11. a	11. d	11. d
12. a	12. b	12. a
13. c	13. d	13. c
14. b	14. c	14. a
15. d	15. a	15. c

Section Test Answers

Test One	Test Two	Test Three	Test Four	Test Five
1. b	1. a	1. b	1. c	1. a
2. d	2. d	2. c	2. d	2. d
3. b	3. c	3. b	3. b	3. c
4. a	4. b	4. c	4. a	4. c
5. c	5. a	5. d	5. c	5. b
6. d	6. c	6. b	6. a	6. c
7. d	7. a	7. a	7. c	7. b
8. a	8. b	8. b	8. b	8. b
9. b	9. c	9. a	9. d	9. d
10. a	10. d	10. b	10. a	10. d
11. b	11. c	11. a	11. c	11. d
12. b	12. b	12. c	12. d	12. a
13. b	13. d	13. c	13. c	13. c
14. a	14. c	14. a	14. a	14. a
15. b	15. b	15. d	15. b	15. b
16. b	16. a	16. a	16. c	16. a
17. d	17. c	17. d	17. a	17. d
18. a	18. b	18. b	18. b	18. a
19. c	19. d	19. b	19. a	19. c
20. d	20. a	20. c	20. c	20. c
21. a	21. c	21. a	21. d	21. c
22. b	22. b	22. c	22. c	22. c
23. d	23. d	23. c	23. c	23. a
24. a	24. b	24. a	24. a	24. c
25. b	25. d	25. b	25. c	25. d
26. c	26. b	26. c	26. d	26. b
27. c	27. d	27. b	27. b	27. b
28. a	28. c	28. c	28. c	28. b
29. c	29. a	29. b	29. a	29. b
30. c	30. b	30. a	30. d	30. d
31. b	31. b	31. b	31. c	31. b
32. a	32. d	32. a	32. b	32. a
33. c	33. c	33. c	33. d	33. a
34. b	34. d	34. c	34. a	34. b
35. d	35. d	35. a	35. d	35. d
36. c	36. a	36. d	36. a	36. a
37. d	37. c	37. b	37. b	37. d
38. c	38. d	38. b	38. d	38. c
39. a	39. b	39. d	39. c	39. d
40. d	40. b	40. b	40. d	40. b
41. c	41. a	41. d	41. b	41. b
42. a	42. b	42. d	42. c	42. c
43. a	43. b	43. b	43. c	43. a
44. b	44. c	44. c	44. d	44. d
45. d	45. d	45. b	45. c	45. d
46. c	46. c	46. c	46. c	46. a
47. b	47. c	47. b	47. b	47. b
48. c	48. b	48. d	48. b	48. b
49. a	49. a	49. b	49. a	49. c
50. a	50. c	50. a	50. b	50. c

Final Examination #1
Answers

1.	a		50.	a
2.	b		51.	a
3.	c		52.	b
4.	c		53.	c
5.	b		54.	a
6.	b		55.	d
7.	a		56.	a
8.	c		57.	c
9.	b		58.	b
10.	d		59.	d
11.	b		60.	d
12.	b		61.	d
13.	d		62.	a
14.	b		63.	d
15.	d		64.	b
16.	b		65.	c
17.	b		66.	c
18.	a		67.	a
19.	d		68.	c
20.	b		69.	d
21.	a		70.	b
22.	d		71.	c
23.	a		72.	a
24.	b		73.	c
25.	c		74.	d
26.	a		75.	a
27.	a		76.	a
28.	a		77.	b
29.	a		78.	a
30.	a		79.	c
31.	b		80.	d
32.	b		81.	d
33.	d		82.	d
34.	a		83.	b
35.	d		84.	a
36.	d		85.	b
37.	d		86.	a
38.	d		87.	b
39.	a		88.	a
40.	c		89.	c
41.	d		90.	a
42.	c			
43.	a			
44.	c			
45.	b			
46.	a			
47.	a			
48.	d			
49.	d			

Final Examination #2
Answers

1. b		52. c	
2. c		53. d	
3. d		54. a	
4. c		55. b	
5. b		56. b	
6. b		57. d	
7. a		58. d	
8. c		59. b	
9. c		60. c	
10. a		61. d	
11. c		62. c	
12. d		63. c	
13. a		64. c	
14. b		65. d	
15. c		66. c	
16. c		67. c	
17. d		68. a	
18. b		69. a	
19. b		70. c	
20. a		71. a	
21. c		72. b	
22. a		73. a	
23. c		74. d	
24. c		75. b	
25. d		76. d	
26. c		77. d	
27. c		78. b	
28. a		79. a	
29. d		80. a	
30. a		81. b	
31. d		82. d	
32. c		83. d	
33. d		84. b	
34. c		85. c	
35. a		86. d	
36. a		87. a	
37. c		88. b	
38. c		89. c	
39. d		90. b	
40. d			
41. c			
42. b			
43. d			
44. a			
45. b			
46. b			
47. d			
48. a			
49. a			
50. d			
51. d			